DIANA JEAN DONALD LIEBISCH

Born in Bogotá, Colombia on September 21, 1961, to a family of Anglo-German ancestry, Diana

studied at the Anglo Colombian School, from where she graduated in 1980.

At the Pontificia Universidad Javeriana she studied Industrial Design, graduating in 1986. In 1987 she married Sergio Loboguerrero. They have three children: Laura (b. 1989), Juan Pablo (b. 1992) and Daniel (b.2003).

Since 1982 she has been suffering from Multiple Sclerosis.

In 2005 Diana and her family moved to Chile, and now live in Puerto Vargas.

In 2008, she had the most severe relapse in her health, which motivated her to write this book.

DIANA JEAN DONALD LIEBISCH

FIGHTING THE IMPOSSIBLE

MULTIPLE SCLEROSIS

I dedicate this book to Sergio, Laura, Juan Pablo and Daniel, for helping me day by day, for being my legs when I lacked them, for helping me with my chores when it was impossible for me to do them, for making me laugh when I was depressed and sad, for giving me strength to fight and get back on the road and for bringing light to my life and meaning to my existence.

PROLOGUE

Two years ago, Diana came into my life, when she was in search for healing and decided to find what she yearned for, in yoga and Sat Nam Rasayan.

At the beginning, she was frail and vulnerable, and as time went by, she became stronger, confronting and starting to fight her illness.

Today I am very happy, because I see that she has found her inner peace and her battle against Multiple Sclerosis became easier.

An illness indicates that an individual has lost order or harmony, that they have lost internal and external balance. Until we learn to see the truths and the facts of this world, we will be tied to our illusions and pain.

We should invite ourselves to step forward into spiritual renewal; as human beings, we will be cured when we find our inner selves. The object of our existence is to become conscious of this, to know ourselves.

This is what Diana has been doing and what she has achieved. This book is witness to her progress and victory facing her illness.

Unfortunately, not many people like her practice the

mind/ body/ soul yoga-union. Only doing a few daily exercises can provide strength, agility, improve circulation, breathing, alleviate stiffness, pain and depression, which help us to be serene, liberating us from conditioning and fear.

Breathing techniques and meditation help us to improve anxiety, anguish, insomnia and stress.

In the long run, these are only a few of the many benefits that are derived from Kundalini yoga. No doubt it has been of great help to Diana. This practice opens us mentally to a new dimension of our existence, in which everything unveils its meaning "and we become Co-creators with God" in the invisible field of the spirit.

Bless this marvellous book, that will be of great help for so many people who are in the daily struggle with their own illnesses.

SAT NAM!

BE EMBRACED BY THE LIGHT

RAVI KAUR KHALSA

KUNDALINI YOGA INSTRUCTOR

SAT NAM RASAYAN

2011

TABLE OF CONTENTS

1. FIGHTING AGAINST THE IMPOSSIBLE

2. THE STORY OF MY LIFE

3. THE DIAGNOSIS OF MY ILLNESS

4. THE FIRST YEARS

5. THE SITUATION IN COLOMBIA

6. THE DIFFICULT REALITY AND THE IMPACT ON MY BODY

7. MY LOSS OF INDEPENDENCE

8. GETTING ADAPTED TO MY NEW PHYSICAL CONDITION

9. LIFE SEEN THROUGH POSITIVE EYES

10. VERY GOOD NEWS: ENTERING THE AUGE PLAN

11. I BEGIN TO INVESTIGATE AND AWAKEN.
A - Water, music and laughter
B - Serotonin and stress
C - Diet
D - The lack of vitamin D.
E - Yoga

12. THE ECONOMIC STRESS

13. THE DEATH OF MY FATHER
F - Breathing

16. DECIDING TO STOP TAKING MY MEDICINE
G - Water divining (dowsing)
H - Healing with the sound of Tibetan bowls and bells
I - Herbal Medicine in Multiple Sclerosis (Phytotherapy)
J - The road to alternative medicine
K - The importance of physical exercise

17. OUR TRAVELING COMPANIONS

18. CONLCUSIONS

AKNOWLEDGEMENTS

Appendix I - MULTIPLE SCLEROSIS DIET

Appendix II - VITAMINS AND SUPPLEMENTS

Appendix III - TWO POSSIBLE ALTERNATIVE THERAPIES DIFFERENT FROM THOSE I USED.

L - Bio-magnetism

M - Acupuncture

REFERENCES

FIGHTING THE IMPOSSIBLE

MULTIPLE SCLEROSIS

1.FIGHTING AGAINST THE IMPOSSIBLE

I am writing this book after fighting with a long illness, which I finally managed to confront and overcome though alternative medicine and the aid of wonderful people, because I want to promote and give strength to other people that are going through situations like mine, show them that they can overcome what in the beginning may seem impossible.

Our mind is so powerful that when we assume a positive attitude in life, facing the pain and the sickness, we promote a series of changes in our body that will help us find the definite improvement and inner peace that we need for healing.

There have been many times in when I have seen my life with negative eyes. Everything covered with black clouds. Every-day life hasn´t been easy. Somehow, I had to overcome certain phases of my illness (Multiple Sclerosis) so I could, with conscious determination, find the way to win the battle.

This book is the recount of my life, my family with

their faults and temperaments, my daily battle, my virtues and faults, my ups and downs, my achievements, and all those moments that have given me the character that I have today and the fortune to defeat an impossible.

Through this narration, I will tell you about the people who have marked my existence positively and whom I call my "guiding lights" because they brought me hope, they gave me the courage and the tools to get ahead when I weakened.

This book is also my token of gratitude to each one of them, for helping me to revive my love for life.

To my three children and Sergio, whom I had given hard times when they were helping me with this illness, I am also deeply grateful to them for they have given me beautiful reasons to live, to stand up, to fight, to raise my head and to walk again, not allowing me to be drowned by this disease.

It was twenty years ago when I was diagnosed with multiple sclerosis, and now, at last, after a series of events during these last two years, I have understood, which road to take for my healing.

Two years ago, I lost the strength in my hands and feet, my balance for walking turned clumsy. I began using a cane and later on a wheel chair. I started to see life in a different way. At the beginning, I cried because I felt impotent and frail, but then I begin my healing process and recovery and that´s when I started writing this book.

2. THE STORY OF MY LIFE

Years ago, when I was starting my way in life, I received the terrible notice of the diagnosis of this difficult, enigmatic and mysterious illness. It felt like I had a time bomb inside me, my world seemed to collapse.

I couldn´t understand it. Why me? Being young and wanting to live, why did I have to confront something like Multiple Sclerosis?

Today, I can say that I am convinced that in our lives there are stages through which we have to pass and a series of events that give us guidance, so that one way or another, we can create our own path, amend our course if we have deflected it and learn to face our destiny. To achieve this, we must accept our condition and ask ourselves, what have we done or not done to be as we are?

Our body is the receptor of everything we do and diseases come when the ground is fertile enough to receive them.

I was born 49 years ago in Bogotá, Colombia in an

English-German family.

I was brought up in a combination of cultures, the tastes of German cooking with the aromas of apple kuchens, chucrut and strudel, along with the strict discipline of the Saxon and the European culture.

I was immersed in the Colombian culture because I lived a great part of my life in Colombia, with its folklore, the typical disorder of a third world country, its food, the arepas, ajiaco, tamales, buns - so many good things, the list will never end. Its merry traditions and spontaneity which made me a mixture of cultures.

Had he been born in another place and time, my father would have been a crazy scientist, for his tireless eagerness in pursuit of learning made him a very prepared person. He had knowledge about everything. He talked about science or politics with the simplicity that characterized him always.

He was always against the corruption in Colombia. He cursed the traffic chaos, losing his patience most times he drove.

Fishing was one of his many hobbies, which always made him feel young. He could spend his time making a perfect fly or a fishing spoon and happily wait for hours by a lake waiting for the miracle of a trout bite.

He was also a radio "ham" and would invest his time trying to communicate with Bangladesh or some other distant place, accumulating contacts and cards from all around the world.

Photography was another of his passions. He built a dark room and developed photographs of our family celebrations. This is where I inherited my love for this hobby.

My parents' friends would joke about my mother never getting anything new for the house, because when something was out of order my father would take it to his workshop. A vacuum cleaner, a phone, whatever, following an easy or complicated surgery, would return better than new.

My mother was always dedicated to her three children. Her artistic side was shown constantly at home, by her watercolours or hand painted porcelain. Seldom do people achieve such simple, delicate and beautiful colour like hers.

She was the head and supervisor of the industry that supported us. Her constant effort and dedication started early in the morning. We could all smell the aromas of maple and corn syrup being prepared in a great pot in the laboratory.

In my teens, I missed out on many things, because my parents hardly let me go out with friends. I attended an elite non-religious British school and my vision of life is radically different to my parents.

However, it was this environment, often difficult to face, that made me strong, adaptable, respectful of the equality between men and women, entrepreneurial and determined to fight. When life gets difficult, we can find the strength we didn´t know we had to achieve our goals.

When we were children, our parents would take us camping on vacations to a beautiful reservoir in the country, north west from Bogotá.

Neusa lake majestically appears in the mist of the Colombian mountains, near plantations of potatoes and onions which scent the countryside.

Little sales tents on the sides of the road offered trout, cheese wrapped in leaves and Colombian sweets. They are attended by the countrymen in their typical ruana (ponchos) and their old hats filled with history, scents and tradition.

Neusa lake was the most economical way to take a vacation once or twice a year. A heavenly place. I remember the mountain as the car would ascend, the colourful little rural houses and the vegetation as we approached the moor, blue, green, violet and grey, until we encountered the beautiful wild plants on the road side, frailejon, trompeto and blackberries.

We had a very nice group of six to eight families that got together taking their children for three weeks a year to Neusa. In later years one of them helped us to get to Chile.

It was a very relaxing time. We would go fishing with hooks and worms, we would hunt for edible mushrooms, for pine cones, swim the freezing water of the lake and its little brooks. We would roll down through the pine forest, had bonfires every night where we would sing (not me because my voice was not the best) play guitar and improvise songs.

It became such a big "family of campers" that we had an annual fair, trout fishing contests and costume parties.

I would practice Olympic gymnastics for hours, because it has always fascinated me. My body was agile, so I could perform all its requirements. I trained every day at the Salitre park in Bogota, had a private instructor and even started an Olympics gymnastics group at school. You need constant training to achieve results, and although I was never "that good", I had a lot of fun and acquired a discipline.

And so I became a teenager and later it was time to go to college. I have always loved design. I think I was born with the gift for this and I was conscious of it. Drawing and photography came very easily to me. I probably inherited this from my parents.

I worked for a year teaching English and managed to enter the university to study Industrial Design.

I moved in with a friend, whose parents were divorced. It was a difficult time for me because I was very lonely, but at the same time my spiritual growth blossomed.

Months later I went back to live with my parents, but now I could go out and live a normal life, like other people of my age.

I have two brothers, the oldest, applied for a post-graduate degree as soon as he could and travelled to the United States, where he got married and settled down. After a few years, he thought of coming back to Colombia, but the panorama of insecurity at that time made him turn in another direction, so he decided to go to Canada.

The youngest is an informatics engineer.

I finished my studies of Industrial Design in the Pontificia Universidad Javeriana. A few months later I met Sergio and within a year we were married.

I met him in one of the most beautiful locations in Colombia, the east planes, at my grandparent's farm on my mother's side, San Antonio, at the exit of the city of Villavicencio.

I went there with friends from my university. The farm wasn´t occupied and at that moment it was available. The farm was one of those old "haciendas", used for cattle, and to be there was like living in another world.

After a long drive leaving Bogota, crossing the east mountain chain, you reach an immense plane, dedicated to livestock, covered with natural grass, rice plantations, African palm and soy. The changes in the temperature are obvious, passing from the cold moor to the medium and intense warm weather of the Llanos plane, where country people still preserve their authenticity.

The aromas of the plants and trees of this warm country float in the air, great areas of plantations flood the horizon, dotted with the intense colour of the farmers' houses.

The house was surrounded by brooks and large trees and the sound of monkeys shrieking, the noise of crickets and cattle at the dawn of the new day.

A livestock farm, which we toured on horseback or walking to the corral where they branded, vaccinated and cleaned long lines of cattle and the workers' camp. We shared lovely stories with them and good local music, called "joropo", which they played on typical instruments, tiple and cuatro (something like small guitars), drinking a glass of a sweet beverage extracted from sugar cane or guarapo (a fermented beverage made of corn or rice). Their cooking, with yuca, banana and chicken broth, with veal or other meats was also delightful.

The house was not free of insects and to avoid further surprises my grandfather built a wall around it, with a small bridge and water under it like a moat, so poisonous snakes, which were very common and many in that area, couldn´t enter.

Nevertheless, you could encounter ugly brown toads at the bottom of the pool or spiders the size of an orange touring the house. Years later Sergio confessed that he fell in love with me when he arrived at the farm and saw me climbing up a mango tree, in my jeans, and tossing the mangos into a basket like a monkey, so we could eat them for lunch.

This is how my life starts hand-in-hand with Sergio, an architect from a family of four brothers, very artistic, hardworking, strong tempered and with fixed ideas. With him I have shared my life for twenty-four years, my struggle with this illness, three wonderful children and my desire to succeed.

We rented a small flat. I started to help him out a little in his office, began selling publicity products, and later commercialised and sold children's clothes with my friend Maria Isabel, whom I had lived with when I left my parent's house.

A few years later our first daughter was born. It seemed like good fortune was knocking at our door. It was a time of a construction boom in Colombia. Our country was wealthy with drug dealing and everyone seemed to want a new house or apartment.

3. THE DIAGNOSIS OF MY ILLNESS

We soon moved to a very spacious house, where our second child was born. Life was giving us beautiful moments, when I began feeling ill.

I felt strange, my hands became numb, my legs froze, my vision blurred. Occasionally I had difficulty swallowing and some days I lost my balance. I thought I was becoming a hypochondriac.

WAS MY MIND PLAYING TRICKS ON ME?

I went from one doctor to another with no results. It was like a game of ping pong in which I was the ball. This ball's hands were numb, feeling unstable, with blurred vision and many strange sensations when waking in the morning.

When my son Juan Pablo was six months old something strange happened. I momentarily lost my vision. it must have been seconds but it seemed like hours. The left side of my body became completely paralyzed... Something was wrong, and now it was serious.

I visited a general doctor, and he sent me to a Neurologist who told me that by the symptoms it seemed that I had a brain tumour.

I have often wondered where some medical professionals get their titles. The damage they can cause with their haste, inexactitude and apparent infallibility is enormous!

After I visited another neurologist, loads of tests were prescribed and the devastating diagnose came: Multiple Sclerosis.

Although I had no idea what this was, I knew it was

serious. My parents took me to the United States for another opinion. I went to the Multiple Sclerosis Association and I learnt how a change in my diet and also alternative medicine could help me.

I decided to cope with it and to concentrate on the part of the glass that was half full, instead of half empty. Our mind is so powerful that if we have a goal, we can achieve it.

4. THE FIRST YEARS

As time passed, I had relapses every twelve to eighteen months, with the same symptoms, numb legs or hands, sometimes the stomach or chest, urgency to find a bathroom, instability, and ending in most cases with a complete recovery.

In the normal transmission of the nervous impulses, a sheath that covers the nerve fibre which improves the transmission plays an important part.

This sheath called *myelin* is produced by important cells of the nervous system called *oligodendrocytes*. The function of the myelin is to ease the transmission of the impulse.

In Multiple Sclerosis (MS) there is an anomalous immunological response that sends some defensive cells of the body (lymphocytes B and lymphocytes T) to a false recognition of strange substances of determined components (called antigens) of the myelin, destroying the myelin sheath (demyelization) and therefore producing an affectation of the signal of the nervous impulses, causing this illness. The loss of myelin can regenerate spontaneously, which happens in the first years of Multiple Sclerosis, forming new sheaths of myelin, which returns the full function to the nervous fibre.

Unfortunately, this process of remyelination, which can be important for some people, may frequently be partial and inadequate and does not fully repair the damage caused previously. Moreover, when the loss of the external sheath is chronic, the nervous fibre suffers damage, leading progressively to inability. That is why, as you age, the aftermath is more visible.

I began to take many kinds of vitamins, followed by a low-fat diet and completely eliminated dairy products from my menu, after reading doctor Roy Lavender Swank's book "The Multiple Sclerosis Diet Book"– a diet, I am sure, helped to keep me relatively well all those years.

The strongest relapse happened in Colombia. We were staying at an old house in a most marvellous town at the old house that belonged to Olguita (my mother in law, who was a widow since she was very young and her second husband, Carlos). Villa de Leyva seemed like a town out of a fairy tale. Villa de Leyva still looks like time stood still. It has Colonial houses with long corridors and patios with geraniums and other beautiful flowers, in the middle of the desert, packed with pimento and olive trees. It's enormous plaza with streets paved in stones, is surrounded with by these beautiful old houses with mud walls, making this a heavenly place.

I started to notice a difficulty in swallowing. The daily insecurity in Colombia and a fright I had a few months before contributed to my stress. When coupled with the property construction recession in Colombia, we decided that it was time to look for a more peaceful place. First, we tried Canada but we never received a visa. I sold the children's clothes stores and I started to work as Director of Cultural at the William Shakespeare Centre in Bogota. It was hard work and there was no weekend rest. I worked until late at night, I had to leave my children who were little and my most precious treasure, my body started to tire and I had frequent relapses, so after three years I thought that this cycle must come to an end, so I resigned and went into the clothes business again.

We mothers always have in our hearts the knowledge of how many children we want to have. In mine, there were always three.

I asked my neurologist if could have another baby and as my other pregnancies had been well and I was in relatively good health, he saw no problem in it.

I started to investigate in the Internet and I found out, after long hours of investigation, that there was an experimental treatment with pregnancy hormones for Multiple Sclerosis sufferers with great results.

I had heard the miracles that the pregnancy hormone can do for Multiple Sclerosis patients and now I am convinced that it is true.

Prolactin levels can provide remyelation and repair the damage in Multiple Sclerosis. Women with Multiple Sclerosis show an improvement of their symptoms during their pregnancy; this is caused by prolactin, which is released by the body in a natural way during pregnancy. A multidisciplinary team has discovered a model of murine experimentation that obtains the reversion of the neural damage in pregnant rats with multiple sclerosis.

(DM. New York 21/02/2007).

The mystery that pregnancy can offer a remission of Multiple Sclerosis comes from a study which shows that a hormone associated with pregnancy is responsible of the reconstruction of the tissue that covers the nerve cells. The results of the study, coordinated by Samuel Weiss, University of Calgary in Canada, and Fred Gage, Salk Institute, San Diego, California, are published in The Journal of Neuroscience.

So we started the pursuit of our third baby. Of course, it is not the same being twenty-seven years old to being thirty-five: now it was somewhat harder to get pregnant again.

Seven years had passed, I was near forty and it was more difficult to think of expecting a third child.

The truth is, I was very anxious and as time passed without conceiving, my anxiety was increasing. On one hand I was conscious of my illness and on the other my advancing age, to the point where I was almost giving up hope. And then I awoke one night from the most marvellous dream a mother can have.

It was a premonition, it really didn´t seem like a dream: a little blue eyed blond boy more or less two years old and he called me mom. I still shiver when I remember this. I woke Sergio up and I told about my dream, although sceptical, he was impressed with the story of my dream. A month later, nature´s miracle became true - I was expecting Daniel.

The miracle I had waited for so many years was now a reality, eight months later I gave birth to a lovely boy whose brother and sister were 11 and 13 years older.

This pregnancy was the most sensational time of my life, with not one symptom of relapse of Multiple Sclerosis.

Daniel brought back our youth. Again, we had a baby at home. It was like going back ten years in our lives. Meanwhile Laura and Juan Pablo were starting High School. Daniel was learning to walk and then going to nursery school. His school mates' parents were obviously much younger than us, which made us feel young again and injected a great dose of energy into our veins.

My sclerosis wasn´t troubling me much, so my neurologist was not in favour of using an immuno-suppressive (for this I will be forever grateful; nowadays very few doctors would do the same). He said I had it under control with the diet and the vitamins. Unwanted secondary effects could appear with a strange medicine, which clearly wasn't a cure, but just a treatment to alleviate the symptoms and a possible prevention to reduce future outbreaks or relapses.

In an effort to produce extra income, we became resourceful and rented our house for film shootings and advertisements. Thanks to a friend we rented our house for films and soap operas, which paid very well. It was like being invaded by aliens running through my house during a very long day.

So, in this way we survived the difficult times we were going through.

5. THE SITUATION IN COLOMBIA

Just like those who have lived all their lives in a violent country like Colombia, we became used to co-existing with violence, kidnapping and delinquency, always thinking that kidnapping happens to others, not to us. Then an important exodus of friends and family began. They were looking for more peaceful countries in which to bring up children. We began to feel isolated, lonely and to suffer in a small amount the fright of living there.

We stopped our usual outings to the country, and fired the workers we knew were related to the guerrilla. We made the decision to leave the country, again seeking peace and security. With the help of my Chilean friend Monserrat Jofré and my younger brother who lived in Puerto Varas, Chile, we managed to move to this beautiful country. Chile received us with open arms.

We left eighteen years of life together behind us and

decided to start life again like two adolescents just beginning to live, but with three children. We didn´t imagine how difficult this would be. We had to start over. What moved us was that our children's future would be different now. We had the possibility of seeing them growing up in a more peaceful country away from the uncertainty we felt in Colombia at that time.

Montse, my Chilean friend and her parents Juan and Ximena, located us in a modest house in Huechuraba. They provided our first needs with such generosity that at that moment of my life I discovered the intrinsic value of the Chileans, their solidarity and commitment to others.

We landed with only what we carried in our hands. Our furniture, memories, and all the little things we accumulate during our lives were left in Colombia waiting to be sent to Chile, once we were settled.

The Jofré family guided us. With such dedication, they held our hand and we took our first steps in this wonderful country. I still remember walking with Montse´s father, clasping his hand. Thanks to him, Sergio started to get around in the city very quickly and a few days later he was completely familiarized with Santiago.

I started to work with Montse, designing and dressing up show cases for shoe stores in all the Santiago Malls and at the same time we offered our services of taking children photographs at schools. And although it was a difficult time for us, since starting up in a foreign country is not easy, even more so when I didn´t have a car during the first year, and I was frequently tired due to the Multiple Sclerosis.

6. THE DIFFICULT REALITY AND THE IMPACT ON MY BODY

The most difficult time of our lives had begun. I was alone here in Chile, with three children, no money and trying to work at whatever came to my reach. Our teenagers were confused and unhappy at having left their country, their home and many memories of their childhood.

Meanwhile in Colombia, Sergio tried to sell our possessions. He worked hard but when he exchanged the devaluated Colombian pesos to Chilean pesos, each Colombian peso became only 25 Chilean cents. After almost a year he was able to return to be with us and start working as an independent architect again.

A short time after our arrival in Chile, my daughter Laura was completely fascinated by her new environment. She spoke like a born Chilean, she even had a boyfriend and said she would never return to Colombia.

I have admired her strong personality, just like her father and I know that any goal she has in life, she will achieve. She is a rebel like I was when I was the same age, with an enormous heart and with an unparalleled fighting spirit.

"The world is in the hands of those who dare to dream and risk living their dreams ": Pablo Coelho.

On the other hand, for my son Juan Pablo this new beginning was more difficult. It seemed that the place where he found himself had little in common with what he had left.

He suffered and went through a lot and during his first year, so much so that when Sergio arrived, we decided to send him to another school. This was the best thing we could have done; the next year, he had wonderful friends and finally was integrated into his new environment.

Juan Pablo is a most noble person, with a sensational personality. God awarded me with such a wonderful human being, so honest, loving and committed (he and Sergio have been my legs since my own went on strike). He wants to learn so many new things, take up so many hobbies and master manual skills, just like my father.

When we travelled to Chile Daniel was two years old. He had no trouble adapting to his new country and today he is more Chilean than Colombian. He is sweet, loving, calm and more outgoing than his brother and sister, so his friends are constantly looking for him. I think he was born under a very special star.

Shortly after Sergio arrived, we decided to move to Chicureo, which in a way it was closer to what we had in Colombia, more like a country life, peaceful and distant from the noise and contamination of Santiago. Juan Pablo's and Daniel's schools were closer to our new home and this made things easier.

I began yoga classes in a wonderful place near our house. I discovered an incredible anti-stress tool and a muscle toner; classes ended with a few minutes relaxation and all this was good for my body and my soul.

Now all these problems and coming to a new country generated additional stress on my weak body and the consequences started with a terrible flu. This in turn awoke my illness, which had been dormant for many years. It resulted in the worst relapse in my life.

The relapse started with difficulty in walking, so I decided it was time to see the doctor again.

After many tests, he decided it was time to begin using immunosuppressants.

Although I wasn't completely in favour of doing so, I started to use Interferon. The daily injection sting was not too difficult to bear, although after a few weeks I felt like a dart board. The funniest thing was that Sergio who has always been fearful of injections, started to sting me with something like a BB gun - the only thing you do is press the trigger and it's done.

But the truth is that our body can't always tolerate certain medications. For each shot, I had to take another medication against side effects. I was taking one medication so the other one wouldn't harm me. You sometimes do things like this when you are desperate.

After a month, I felt worse than I was when I started the treatment so after the third month, when I could hardly walk, I decided 'No More Shots'. I preferred to stay as I was.

But the damage was done. One day as I was driving from Santiago and one of my legs went on strike. I was so scared. I managed to take control of the car and I parked until my leg was normal. Fortunately, I was safe, but I decided to stop driving because I was afraid an accident could happen. Now I would have to depend more on Sergio to get me around.

7. MY LOSS OF INDEPENDENCE

I could do practically nothing. Even the simplest things like bathing or getting dressed became very difficult. It really wasn´t a good time, it was like living a nightmare and I prayed to God to help me get out of it.

Sergio had to do the chores I once did, like driving and picking up the children from school, or going to the supermarket. Simple things, but they took up a lot of his time.

My neurologist suggested switching to another medicine and so I started Copaxone. This is a glatimer acetate, a protein which simulates the effects of the basic protein of myelin, indicated for reducing the frequency or seriousness of patients with remittent multiple sclerosis, as is my case. It was a radical change, with no collateral side effects. The problem was its very high cost. I don´t think even a millionaire could keep up paying one million Chilean pesos a month. After one year of treatment, we couldn´t afford paying for it any longer. I stopped taking the drug, fearful and certain that I would get worse every day. At least, that was what I expected.

At this point my first "guiding light" appears. I had to have a pastime or else I would go crazy, so I stated ceramic classes, which from the beginning proved to be the best therapy I could have chosen. My weak and awkward hands couldn't help me very much, but the therapy of the "copucha" (that is how talking with friends - "gossip" - is called here in Chile) and getting away from home for a while, was very useful.

A few months later I was granted a scholarship. It was obvious that I couldn't pay for extra classes. Bea, my teacher and my first "guiding light" helped me out, without knowing, in recovering my self-esteem and my desire to continue the struggle. I would rush to her house knowing it would be a morning of relaxation. With her dedication helping me to take steps forward, her lovely positive attitude and generosity, she gave me the urge to survive, which wouldn't have happened if I hadn't met her in that exact moment. The result of these classes: my soul recovered overwhelming strength.

In Indian religions, there are four spiritual laws:

The first one is: *The person that comes is the right person, no one comes into our lives accidentally.*

The second is: *What happens was meant to be happen. Nothing, absolutely nothing occurs in our lives, that could have happened in any other way.*

The third is: *What happens at any time, it's because it is the right moment, not before, not after.*

The fourth is: *When something ends, it ends. If something ends in our lives, it is for our evolution, so the best thing is to carry on.*

The simplest house work became more and more difficult and easy things turned into very slow work, almost impossible for me to do. It's hard to believe that with the blink of an eye, your obedient body stops being so and we become dependent and vulnerable.

I began using a cane. My neurologists advised that I needed something to aid me, because my stability was low and the risk of falling was high. To begin with, it was difficult to accept that I couldn't depend on my own legs and that people would see me as a handicapped person, but in the end I told myself: It's better to see a "handicapped" person in one piece than a "stubborn" person in many pieces and the cane became my everyday companion.

There were days when I choked and my throat wouldn't accept meals. I felt helpless and miserable, thinking that in one or two years I wouldn't be able to eat at all and would be entering the ranks of the vegetative beings.

But that was not the worst. I was thinking of the horror it would be for Sergio to help a person in that condition and even sadder not to see my children growing up, not to share helping them with their homework, not cooking something special for eating together or walking with them in a lovely day of summer. And in the end, to be there with them in their achievements and lift them in their falls.

My desperation was such that I wrote a good-bye letter, telling them how fortunate I had been to be able to share precious years of my life with them. I still keep that letter and fortunately I never had the courage to deliver it.

I travelled to Colombia to try another treatment that looked promising in helping MS. It was with a crazy scientist who was also a veterinarian. The consultation took place in the veterinarian office and I waited in the company of his normal patients: a Rottweiler and a Poodle. He said he had the cure for MS, but after a month and a half of hearing of parasites that released toxins in your system and treatments for these, that supposedly were responsible for Multiple Sclerosis, nothing was achieved. Only my visit to my homeland and a good bye to my father, who died a short time after.

My daughter Laura had been to Colombia on vacations and when she saw her school friends, her heart was telling her to stay where she was born and with her friends. She renewed her culture and the traditions she was brought up with. She decided not to return to Chile and to continue her studies in Colombia, living with her grandmother.

8. GETTING ADAPTED TO MY NEW PHYSICAL CONDITION

Back to the daily routine again, the lack of money was our Achilles heel. We were behind in every payment. Trying to buy the Multiple Sclerosis medicine during almost a year cased our finances to go into a spin. The global recession didn´t help either.

Economic conditions can reduce human beings to a constant level of stress and if a family member is ill, this situation can easily generate into complete financial chaos.

Life was becoming more and more difficult and with every day that passed, my frail body lost strength and I had less desire to struggle. We could not afford my medicine and psychologically I became more vulnerable.

Everyday chores became a complete odyssey for me. I was more and more restricted and lonely. It was at this moment when a series of promising events began. Little by little they brought back my hope and the strength to continue my struggle.

Our friends became very important for us. Their invitations, their gay spirits and solidarity made us feel at home. These friends became part of our family in such way that we didn´t feel alone. They are my second "guiding light". They encouraged my wanting to get ahead again, not to give up, not to sink into sadness and disability in my daily struggle with this illness.

"You only succeed in this world if you get up and seek for the circumstances and make them happen if you don´t find them ": George Bernard Shaw.

By September, our economic situation was worse, so Sergio and I decided to sell some of the antique rugs we had in order to pay a few debts, especially health insurance which we hadn´t paid in almost a year. Because of this I wasn´t able to return for medical check-ups.

We called several art galleries, and one of them caught our attention, so the next day we went to the owner. When we arrived, she asked us to enter her office. She asked me why I was limping. I told her I had Multiple Sclerosis and she looked astonished. A friend of her daughter who also had Multiple Sclerosis had gone to healing masses and had immediately been cured.

"Why don´t you try it?" she said.

I didn´t want to go through what happened weeks before when Dani asked me:

-       Mom   Does   God   exist?

- Of course, Dani. Why?

- If he exists, where does he live?

- In heaven, Dani.

- Oh, I understand. And is it above or below the Martians?

The truth is, I didn´t know where God would be at that

moment, because I didn´t feel him close to me. I think Dani was right and he must have been with the Martians at that moment, but I am a Catholic, a believer, although not very observant. I have seen many people go to church to seek forgiveness and later continue to be the same selfish and egocentric persons they were before, without practicing what they heard the preacher say.

But at this time of my life, I had nothing to lose so I asked her to give me more information and two weeks later I went with Sergio to this healing mass. it was an old church in the centre of Santiago, cold, smelling strongly of damp, and a little melancholic, but there I found absolute peace. in that afternoon, I felt that something had touched my soul, beyond finding a cure. I cried as I had never done before and I couldn´t stop my tears. They flowed through an open door that couldn´t be closed. Hundreds and thousands of tears came out or my eyes, but at the end I felt peaceful and found a different way to face my problem and my life.

That day I decided to fight against everything.

They say that a positive attitude brings us many solutions and this is precisely what began to happen with me.

9. LIFE SEEN THROUGH POSITIVE EYES

On September 23, the owner of the gallery called again to let us know she had sold our rugs. This is the way that the miracle of healing started. Without her knowledge, she gave me new hope in my daily struggle. We could pay what we owed to our health insurance, so I was calmer with regards to my illness.

Eight days later I had to go shopping. Sergio had gone to work. So I decided to call a cab and looking for a card, I found the number of a driver I had called a year before. I called him. He arrived twenty minutes later. I couldn't anticipate what was going to happen that afternoon, how he would impress me and make me react to the story he told me.

He arrived very well dressed. I entered the cab with my two children, with certain difficulty trying to place my cane in the rear of the cab.

After explaining the route to him, he very politely asked me:

"Why are you limping? Were you in an accident? "

I said no, I have Multiple Sclerosis and I had a relapse two years ago and since then I have been lame and can´t walk well.

"What is that?" he asked me.

I explained to him that it was a neurologic demyelating, neurodegenerative and chronic sickness of the central nervous system, something like peeling the electric wires that are in our brain, which causes a limited mobility or invalidity in severe cases, vision problems and many other things.

I saw his face through the driving mirror and how interested he was with my explanation.

Soon he turned back and asked me:

"Could you let me know more? I´m interested in knowing more and I will tell you why later".

I explained further, giving him more explanations about the topic, telling him about how and when it started and the different symptoms I've had during these last seventeen years.

We continued on our route and seldom have I seen such an efficient worker, not only as a cab driver, but a guide ready to help in any way. Twenty minutes must have passed when he told my children that they had to help me in everything, because it was obvious that I couldn´t do the work I had done before and had difficulty in walking.

Juan Pablo and Daniel would dismount at every place we arrived, did the shopping we needed and would return to the cab.

Soon the driver began to tell me he understood my condition, because his wife had pancreatitis. She was given no hope in surviving but miraculously she was alive and that he was sure it was her determination that saved her, because he refused to disconnect her from the machines that kept her alive.

Now she is well with only a few limitations.

We finished our shopping and we started to go back home. He still continued talking to the children about the importance of helping me. When we arrived home, I paid him, he got out of the car and helped me out. He gave me his card. After he left I looked at it and read:

DON´T ASK GOD

TO SOLVE YOUR PROBLEMS

ASK HIM TO GIVE YOU THE STRENGTH TO FACE THEM.

A weird chill overwhelmed me that afternoon.

Why in that exact moment did that card turn up?

That afternoon I reaffirmed my decision that I was going in the right direction, to think positive, because with positive thoughts you build the road.

As Norman Cousins tells us in his multiple investigations on the power of laughter, the most important thing is your attitude towards your illness.

His scientific study rendered obsolete the theory of the central nervous system and the systems that control the endocrine and immunologic functions as being separate. All those positive elements, like love, hope, faith, desire to live, determination, purpose and laughter, they avoid depression and aid the healing process of your body.

A few days ago, I went to the healing mass to ask God to heal me of Multiple Sclerosis so I could start walking again, when I should have asked for strength in facing my illness and return to positive thinking.

My mind began this miraculous process and this brought many good things that I had been seeking for many months.

A few days later and thanks to the help of friends in Chile I was able to renew my treatment which I had to discontinue a year ago, due to its cost. I really don't know if it was good to restart it, but it was a part of my life I had to seal.

I started to take Copaxone and psychologically, I think that now I began to feel stronger and more determined to win the battle.

10. VERY GOOD NEWS: ENTERING THE AUGE PLAN

Multiple Sclerosis was accepted in the Auge Plan, which meant that my medication, beginning 2010, is covered by the government. We owe this great achievement to Claudia Opazo and to the group of patients and their families who dedicated many hours in public demonstrations and efforts with authorities and politicians to make this happen.

Santiago, November 13 - The Multiple Sclerosis group of Patients expressed their approval to the official announcement of the Ministry of Health concerning the entry of this neurodegenerative pathology to the Auge Plan, beginning next year in July.

"In 2008, the approval of both chambers of Congress included the incorporation of this illness to the Auge Plan. Thanks to this and the efforts of Senator Soledad Alvear (DC) and the minister of Health, Alvaro Erazo, it was possible to enter the General Regime of Guarantees, which allowed that the treatment of this pathology would count with the Fonasa coding system ". Source: UPI

11. I BEGIN TO INVESTIGATE AND AWAKEN

A - Water, music and laughter

A few months ago, I heard about the benefits of water and it's healing power. I began to investigate more and more about the fascinating world of water, the discoveries of Masaru Emoto, graduate in International Relations and later in alternative medicine, who began to study the healing properties of water. He also contacted an investigator in California who studied the molecular vibrations of water, using the technique of magnetic resonance.

Emoto asked himself if it would be possible to reflect the healing properties of different types of water in a visible and tangible way.

He took photographs of the hexagonal crystals which form in the water when it froze. With these images, he confirmed his hypothesis:

"Some samples of running water in big cities showed crude crys-

tallization structure, while water from brooks showed crystals of great beauty. "

He extended the area of his studies, taking photographs of water from different parts of the world (glaciers, lakes, rain water, fountains), obtaining more beautiful and amazing shapes the more distant they were from human contamination.

The biggest surprise came when he managed to transform irregular patterns of contaminated water into beautiful hexagonal crystals by submitting the samples to the sound of traditional music, religious prayers or classical music.

He managed to transform 'indifferent' crystals of distilled water into lovely geometric patterns when he whispered words of gratitude to them and, conversely, obtaining distorted structures when saying harsh words to the water.

If we human beings are basically water, can we get the same results?

As Santiago Rojas describes it in his book "The strategy of the Phoenix Bird": "...something like being allergic to your own body". As the immune system responds directly to our thoughts and feelings, so our nutrition should begin by loving ourselves, and taking care and respect of our selves.

The exercises of creative imagination - like our inner happiness - are ideal for giving the best feelings to all our body.

I continued investigating so intensely. I couldn´t stop reading new books and searching the internet, finding each time more and more astonishing and interesting results, which I had skipped for many years. Maybe sometimes you have to reach the end of the tunnel to start finding your way out.

Doctor F. Batmanghelidj, M.D. describes the following statements in his book: *"Every function of your body is regulated by and depends on water. Water is necessary for carrying vital elements, oxygen, hormones and chemical messengers to all the body. Without enough water to humidify the body, probably some remote parts won´t receive the vital elements water could have given them. Water is also necessary for expelling toxic waste from the cells. You can recover memory, even in old age, the brain is 85% water. When it lacks water, it shrinks. The cells, normally shaped like rounded grapes, become raisins. The investigation shows that Alzheimer disease occurs when chronic dehydration has affected the brain cells. When they dehydrate, many body cells die. Other cells of the body produce new cells; that does not happen in the brain, they are not replaced".*

If the investigations of doctor Emoto concluded that with just changing the music and talking quietly to water, it promoted a radical change in its structure, I thought I have to begin speaking to my body positively.

Would I be able to transform the irregular water patterns of my body responsible for my illness, into the beautiful crystals that would aid it in healing and reverse my actual condition?

Would I need to provide my system with more water, like doctor F. Batmanghelidj proposed?

It was evident that during the last two years I didn´t drink enough water, so I started to increase gradually the amount of water I drank, so my body wouldn´t become one of the "raisins group"- like Daniel said to me with the ingenuity that only a child has: "When I grow old, Mum, will I be an ugly and wrinkled old man or is that not going to happen to me?"

Unfortunately, it will happen to all of us but at least it will take a little longer if we take enough water. The problem for those with MS is that if we drink much water, we risk not getting to the bathroom on time, because one of the symptoms of Multiple Sclerosis is urinary incontinence.

Would Multiple Sclerosis (characterized by an alteration of the immune system) act against my own cells as if they were harmful agents simply because of the stress or tension to which I have been under these last two years?

For not having the conviction that I was going to win the battle and instead thinking every day that I had already lost it and I was defeated?

During the next weeks, I began to make different daily experiments with my body. Anyone that saw me would think it was a severe case of madness. I would do this while the children and Sergio were out, so I was completely peaceful and alone and no one could interrupt me. I also didn´t want them to see me doing all these mad things:

I began listening to relaxing melodies, like those which Emoto used to get beautiful patterns in the water:

Imagine,   John   Lennon

REM, Everybody hurts

Sting, Until

Israel Kamakawiwo, In this life

Israel Kamakawiwo, Sea of love

Jack Johnson, Breakdown.

And many others. I repeated them all morning and by noon I would analyse how I felt and I would constantly repeat to myself: Courage, it can be done, I can win this battle.

I began to notice that the softer the music, the more peaceful I felt. It was easier to walk in the afternoon and as I had more positive thoughts I would feel much better.

During the day, I laughed about everything and I also noticed that for many years my body had acquired that helping release. When I had a tense moment, I would laugh. Even when I corrected my youngest child I couldn´t help laughing, in the end with mixed emotions.

What could a six-year-old child think about when this strait faced mother, in the middle of scolding him, would burst out in laughter?

The advantage is that laughter is free medicine.

"Laughter is a muscular exercise that moves great parts of the muscles of the body: abdominals, facial, limbs. It acts on the respiratory axis, dilating bronchia and increasing the amount of air you breathe.

It is a cardiovascular stimulator, it lowers blood pressure and decreases heart rate. Improves the digestion, it's a therapeutic massage of the bowels, increases the bowel movements and combats constipation. Laughter releases cerebral endorphins, acts against pain and increases secretion of serotonin. A depressed person has low levels of serotonin. It acts upon the neuro vegetative system, decreases stress and encourages sleep. It is a psychic stimulant. " Luz Adriana Neira – Maria Ninelly Neira - Doctor Clown Foundation 1999. Colombia.

B - Serotonin and stress

"We live in times in which we know that stress affects sickness more and more, so why don't we do something about it?" Joan Borysenko MD: "YOUR MIND CAN CURE YOU."

I decided to get stress out of my life so I tried to get away from the constant problems of my family and look for shelter with my "Chilean family ". My pottery classes became more precious to me. They were my weekly therapy. They made me happy, something like group therapy for laughing, in order to face life by changing my way of thinking, from negative to positive.

My emotional state and perception of life began to transform, thanks to the happiness and optimism I was encountering.

I found out that to be calm and to try to remove depression - the daily companion of my life - I had to regulate my serotonin. Serotonin are neurotransmitters which are located in different parts of the central nervous system and have great influence on our moods.

The increase of serotonin in nervous circuits produces a sensation of well-being and relaxation.

Among its functions:

- It regulates our appetite through satiation, regulates sexual urge, controls body temperature, motor activity and perceptive and cognitive functions.

- It involves other known neurotransmitters like dopamine, noradrenalin, which are related to anguish, anxiety, fear, aggressiveness, and also eating problems.

- It is necessary to develop melatonin, a protein made by the brain in the pineal gland and is responsible of regulating sleep. Serotonin, increasing toward the evening, induces sleep and continues at elevated levels until dawn, when it declines.

- It acts like the inner clock of our body, which determines our sleep patterns. The internal clock is in charge of the coordination of several biologic functions, like body temperature, stress hormone, cortisol and sleep patterns. The correct coordination of these three elements makes us have deep sleep and wake up rested. Men produce up to 50% more serotonin than women, therefore women are more sensitive than men to changes in serotonin levels.

Why does the level of serotonin change?

Stress, levels of sugar in the blood and hormone changes, of which oestrogen is the most important, are some of the factors that alter the serotonin level.

Serotonin can be measured in a blood test, although not completely, because the brain and the rest of the body are separated by a brain hemi-barrier - a kind of shade that will not admit the passing of a strange substance to the brain. That is why the brain has its own neurotransmitters.

How to increase that marvellous hormone, that I felt I needed?

Tryptophan is the precursor of serotonin. This essential amino acid can trespass the cerebral barrier, and must be obtained through a diet.

Techniques of relaxation, yoga, and meditation help to boost the serotonin levels.

Regular exercise, fresh country air, travel and dance also help.

The change of activities, doing new things, starting projects, travelling.

C - Diet

The question then, was obvious.

What food should I begin to eat?

We have always heard that there is nothing better than good feeding. Our ancestors knew how to cure through nature and the right food but we somehow lost all this wisdom.

Why is it that in this century, depression is one of the most extended ailments of humankind?

Why have so many new diseases appeared?

Could it all be caused by an improper diet that increases the levels of stress in society?

It is very easy to find everyday someone that will tell us that they are passing through a difficult depressive state. The effects can be devastating. Depression is the main reason that people go to a psychoanalyst and psychotherapists.

But could we alleviate all this simply with a change of attitude toward ourselves?

There are two miracle fruits that contain certain special amino acids that stimulate the happiness hormone (serotonin). They have fascinating properties that combat many maladies, including Multiple Sclerosis:

Banana: Besides fighting against depression, it helps digestion and reduces bad cholesterol in the blood. Its content of carbohydrates is high, hence it's caloric value is high. Banana´s highest nutrients are potassium, folic acid and astringent substances; it also provides a great amount of oligosaccharide type fibre.

Potassium is a necessary mineral for the transmission and generation of the nervous impulse and also for muscular activity, and it intervenes in the water balance in and outside the cell. Magnesium is related with the bowel function nerves and muscles. It forms part of bones and teeth, improves immunity and provides a gentle laxative. Folic acid intervenes in production of red and white blood cells; in short, the genetic material and formation of the antibodies of the immune system. It contributes in preventing anaemia and spina bifida in pregnancy.

Potassium is a vital mineral that helps to regulate heart beats, sends oxygen to the brain and regulates the water balance of the body. When we are stressed, our metabolic rate increases and reduces our level of potassium.

Melon: Should always be consumed ripe. When you press the ends and they sink a little, it is ripe. Besides combating depression, melon has a gentle laxative effect and protects the stomach. It is a diuretic, it eliminates the toxins of our body.

D - The lack of vitamin D.

I also discovered that my sclerosis got worse when I changed countries, from Colombia to Chile. Something in the environment had changed in a radical way. For fifteen years, my sclerosis was quite controlled in Colombia and it was only in these last two years in Chile that it decided to trouble me with more impetuosity.

What did I have in Colombia and had lost with the change of countries?

When I began investigating, what I found out was overwhelming. It was the lack of vitamin D.

Why do parts of Canada, the north of the United States and Scandinavian countries have higher rates of Multiple Sclerosis?

The answer to this question has given initiative to exploration for new treatments for this illness.

"It has been observed that in the places where there is a lower incidence if solar light there is a higher incidence of the malady. This could be because the inhabitants of those places have

lower levels of vitamin D (which is produced by the skin when it is exposed to sun light)", said Doctor Jorge Correlale, neuro-immunological chief of Fleni, that published a study that explains why the deficiency of vitamin D is associated with greater risk of Multiple Sclerosis.

"This opens the possibility of using vitamin D as a tool for part of the treatment ", says Correale, and also that the right dosage is still to be determined so it won´t have undesired side effects.

Correale went one step further and studied the relation of different elements of the immunological system to find how the deficiency of vitamin D is associated with inflammatory phenomena characteristic of Multiple Sclerosis.

In MS, the communication between the brain and other parts of the body is interrupted. Many experts believe that it is an auto immune sickness in which the body, through a defence system, attacks its own tissues.

Vitamin D inhibits the growth of the cells that destroy myelin (which covers the nerves), blocks the liberation of pro-inflamatory substances (citoquinas) and increases the number of regulating cells that block the toxic action of the cells that destroy myelin.

"All these protective effects of the nervous system disappear when there is a deficiency of vitamin D" (Sebastian A. Rios, LA NACION).

E - Yoga

New people came to our weekly pottery weekly class. One of them practiced yoga and specifically the technique called Sat Nam Rasayan. This is a method of relaxation and healing that teaches one how to liberate tendencies and limitations of the body, mind and spirit. It showed me a new horizon of hope and healing through yoga. The interior silence is considered by all the traditions of meditation as the highest peak of achievement.

This technique teaches an advanced way of reaching and sustaining that interior silence under all the and stress of daily life.

Sat Nam Rasayan stabilizes the energy flow of a person. My pottery friend spoke to me about it and I was very interested in the topic. It was, in a way, what I been looking for during all this time: a return to yoga. She told me that a friend of hers, Ravi, was specialised in yoga healing. She asked her friend not to charge me for the consultation because I needed the therapy but at the moment I had no way of paying for it. As miracles happen, Ravi received me for my first Sat Nam Rasayan therapy two weeks later.

Ravi became my third "guiding light ". She gave me strength and the inner peace necessary for healing.

My arrival to my first yoga therapy came with a halo of suspense. Really I didn´t know what I was going to do there. Ravi lives near Escuela Militar subway station, in a building where I had to exit down a staircase. For a person who trips easily this is an obstacle. Fortunately, Sergio came with me and helped me to her door.

I rang the bell and the door was opened by a large woman, big of body and soul, wearing a white turban and long robe, with a kind and peaceful voice, irradiating peace and calm.

I entered a room and laid down on a bed. During the first half hour, I talked to her about my life through my childhood up until now.

She wrote down on a pad all the details necessary for my healing. Then she turned on soft music and told me to close my eyes and to take deep breaths, inhaling and exhaling very slowly. She placed her hand on my left arm and began the healing process for more than an hour. When I finally opened my eyes, I felt great peace. She then told me about mantras and how to use them day by day, also the importance of breathing.

Mantras are sounds that connect us with different levels of intelligence. Sat Nam is the basic mantra used in Kundalini yoga. Sat means truth, Nam is name, identity. Sat Nam can be translated as "the Truth is the name of God. The truth is my (your, our) identity".

It is used like a greeting to recognize the truth in each of us and like a personal mantra to express or to tune in to the infinite identity of one's self.

But exactly what is the Sat Nam Rasayan?

The patient lies down on a bed and the healer places their hands on the patient's arm and leaves them motionless. The healer then enters a state of deep meditation. Patient and healer remain in absolute silence and after half an hour the healer withdraws their hands.

Both healer and patient remain in a deep state of tranquillity; the patient feels a greater energy and peace. In theory, the blockage that existed disappears and the malady will begin to improve.

The healer limited herself to the practice of a very ancient healing technique called Sam Nam Rasayan, which has extraordinary results.

What happens in that half hour of silence and immobility?

We seem to be in the presence of a wizard, or a great healer gifted with extraordinary powers.

The truth is that anyone could learn Sat Ram Rasayan. The great achievement of Guru Dev Singh, master of this technique, was to design a system that allows any person to learn it, simply by application and constant practice.

In the yoga healing, the only instrument of healing is the consciousness of the healer, who reaches a state of meditation, from where he/she induces changes in the patient.

It was time to get back to being productive. I have always believed that activity is good for us. Leisure is the worst thing that could happen to a person who is fighting against illness, because it gives you time to feel sorry for yourself.

I renewed my writing of children stories with the idea of getting them published. I worked on Graphic Design, trying to start a business with some friends so I could help out with expenses. Little by little I began to get excited with all this and I began to feel productive again.

12. THE ECONOMIC STRESS

Our economic situation at this time was chaotic, but good friends and near ones made this difficult moment an enriching economic experience. It showed us the meaning of solidarity and helping a person in need when it is required.

Tomas Cox, Patricia Ready and Jaime Fuenzalida are my fourth "guiding light ". They "put on their shirts " so they could help us find our way out of this situation. To put on your shirt means to help others, that is the how they say it in Chile. "Apechugar "is not easy, it is hard work, dedication and generosity.

They set out to help us solve many of our economic problems, which were causing terrible and uncontrollable additional stress to our daily living and therefore a constant damage to my illness. You can´t heal physically if you don´t ease the external burden generated by stress.

I owe them for helping me to recover peace, thanks to their endless efforts and generous unselfish aid. Through their contacts, we managed to pay off most of our debts. With it, I removed that endless stress from my life which had seemed impossible to do.   The incredible part of this is that people who we had met recently in a foreign land were much more caring than my own family.

Nobody likes having debts, but sometimes we go through difficult times in our lives. We hadn't imagined that an illness can be so devastating. No normal family finances can cope with that high price, on top of which we were in a strange country with limited contacts and suffering more than a headache. We had to learn from it, to grow and be better persons.

13. THE DEATH OF MY FATHER

My daughter Laura informed me about my father´s health. He was very ill. It was very clear at that moment that the condition of my health would make it very difficult to travel to Colombia alone, with all the inconveniences of airports, walking, customs etc.

The reality was that if my father was dying I couldn´t travel to bid him a final good bye.

Sad as I was. I decided to write him a letter, to be read by my daughter Laura at his funeral as my farewell to him:

"My dear Patico (Duck, that´s the way his friends called him because his surname was Donald).

Only God knows how much I would have wanted to be with you to say good bye and thank you for everything you taught me since my childhood.

There are times in our lives when we can´t be where we want, but that does not mean that in my heart I am not with you. A year ago, when I came back from a holiday in Colombia to Chile, you were holding my hand and you said you would miss me very much. I knew somehow that it was our final good bye.

Today I want to remember all the things that will be in my memory forever and how I am so proud that I came into this world because of you.

The memories of our dear Neusa with its fishing, the aroma of pine trees and damp moss, the walks looking for wood, the nights with the campfire and the hunts for berries where we felt like explorers, will remain with us as a memory of our childhood.

Your workshop, your radio, your Scots melodies, your unending pastimes like airplane modelling and photography, will remain in our hearts like a very special legacy for our children.

A million words can´t bring you back.

Nor a million tears.

I say good bye from the bottom of my heart

I say goodbye forever, although you will be in my memory.

Your daughter Diana".

In the morning of December second I received the phone call I feared. It was my daughter Laura telling me my father had died.

Our parents are the pillars of a building that we slowly build as the years go by; they give us all at the beginning of our life when we are vulnerable, they help us to be who we are when we are older and then they in turn become vulnerable and old, almost without notice, solitary and dependent on us.

Something strange coincided with his death. Patricia Ready the lady owner of the art gallery, met Thomas Cox, who told her about our situation, to see how things could be sold faster. She sent us the financial help we never expected. In these moments, we see how miracles exist and happen. Miracles are carried out every day by wonderful people like them.

I received a call informing me that they will buy one of the sculptures we were selling. It was as if something coming from the afterlife was giving us a wonderful gift. My father had just died and the universe expressed itself as if the voyage he had undertaken just a day before was helping us. Now we could pay almost all our debts.

The God that in some moment was keeping company with the Martians (like my son Daniel used to say) was here with us and was a reality.

They told me my father´s funeral mass was very quiet and sad, with all the people that wanted to say their last farewell. The letter I sent him from the bottom of my soul was read by my daughter and with it I eased my mind for not being able to travel.

When someone so intelligent and cultured departs, it is very sad. With him also leaves all the knowledge he acquired during a lifetime. My father was a wandering encyclopaedia; he knew about everything and what he didn´t know, he investigated. My British encyclopaedia left with him, the encyclopaedia of my life.

It was December, Christmas was near, so I decided to ask my friend Bea, who was a friend, more a sister for me, to come to the mall to shop for a few things. To make it easier for me, she asked for a wheelchair so I could move around and it was the first time I remember requesting one. Maybe I didn't want to recognise limitations but it was the best help I could have and now I use it frequently because I tired after fifteen minutes and couldn't see a thing. This way we could shop and there was time for coffee – tintico, like we say in Colombia.

I kept going to the clinic every month for the cortisone shots. That way they would give me the Multiple Sclerosis medicine. I wasn´t too sure that I was doing the right thing. Submitting my body to cortisone without a reason couldn´t have been very good, since a few days after I would feel a tremendous lack of strength.

My yoga sessions, Sat Nam Raysan began to be a benefit for my health. I discovered that due to all the stress I had coped with this year had blocked my breathing and my oxygenation had diminished considerably, so one of the things I did was to practice how to improve it.

F - Breathing

Breathing is a fountain of health. It guarantees the strengthening our body and our mind. Most of us don´t breathe correctly; we do it superficially. as if we were afraid of what breathing can do.

Yoga breathing covers 3 parts of the body.

Abdominal, where it starts.

Intercostal, where it continues.

Thoracic or clavicular, where it is supposed to finish the process of inspiration.

At the beginning, as we are not used to conscious breathing. When we arrive at the intercostal zone we don´t have breathing capability, so our inspiration cannot reach the thoracic zone, but with practice we can increase that capacity.

The rhythm should be slow and smooth, the breathing must start in the abdominal zone and with a slow lifting, it continues spreading the inspiration towards the "intercostal" zone. You should feel your ribs opening and moving to the sides, continuing up to the thoracic zone.

Breathing is essential for our body, we must breathe deeply to provide energy. It automatically produces a peaceful sensation if done correctly and slowly enough. it also regulates the pH (acid-alkali) balance in our body and this affects our reactions in stress situations, increases the "prana", the oxygen making us more alert and conscious. It cleans and purifies the blood, and allows the brain to make the right decision in critical situations. The good perform-ance of the body's electromagnetic field depends on the complete use of pulmonary capacity, reduces the accumu-lation of toxins in the lungs, stimulates the production of substances that help combat depression, reduces fear and the anxiety, eliminates blockages in the energy flow and cleans energetic channels.

14. A POSITIVE ATTITUDE

I´m firmly convinced that, independent from physical healing, emotional healing is even more important. It not only helps our body to have enough energy to struggle against our illness, but it also gives us something even more important, the will to strive and go forward. This is distinct from the physical difficulties we might have, caused by the damage or progress of our illness.

To achieve this and in accordance with what I have been through these years, this is a topic on our attitude towards life and how we should cope with our illness. I feel that I have healed emotionally and in order to defeat the battle against my physical illness, this is the most important part. I don´t know if I will be able to walk again, but I am calm and I know that I will do my best in pursuing it. The universe will be in charge of making the rest possible.

My yoga sessions have been fundamental for my healing. In my first therapies with my "healer" she showed me two spheres of different colours. One, she said, is the negative thoughts, the other the positive thoughts. Both will be present in every moment of your life. The negative will remain as long as we let it. We can only heal through our own experience, getting through a state of consciousness in which we set aside all these negative thoughts. Our own body is capable of being our own healer; we have the power to do it; we only have to give our own energy the opportunity of helping us to achieve it.

Focusing the energy on the different parts of our body is the most wonderful of the yoga exercises. Starting with the tip of the toe and ending in our brain, the highest part of our body, we notice how each part of the body nurtures on it and how the miracle of this sensation can emanate from us.

The question arises again, how much beneficial can the treatment I am receiving with the Copaxone and the Cortisone be? It doesn't cure or decrease the symptoms of Multiple Sclerosis, but it is supposed to be very efficient at stopping the evolution of the illness, by as much as a 30%.

I can only see the desire of some laboratories to convince us that it is beneficial (for their pockets), but not for our health. I am in much pain and lack of strength when I leave the clinic, because they have turned us into the most profitable business on the planet.

As Ghislaine Lanctot rightly says in her book "The Medical Mafia."   Many of the maladies that are nowadays chronic have a cure, but it's not profitable to cure them in their totality.

Lanctot came fast to a conclusion that non-aggressive medicine is more effective, cheaper and has less side effects.

Doctors constantly travel to conventions all over the world, to learn about the recent medical advances.

But who finances those conventions?

Big laboratories and the Pharmaceutical industries. *"The medical career is first of all a business."*

To keep the control and continue to be profitable, they

have to ensure that the patients remain patients.

"Healthy people don´t produce income, while sick people do."

The trick is to keep us as chronic patients, so we consume all kinds of products to treat our symptoms, but in the long run these don´t cure us.

It's a system that keeps us dependant and at the same time, stimulates us to consume drugs of all types.

The doctors re-transmit to their patients the great advances in medicine of the laboratories and without knowing it they become the laboratories' puppets, but in the eyes of we 'the patients', they are like a generation of God's carriers of the latest medical news.

It´s easy to make a simple calculation:

In Chile, there are 3,000 people with Multiple Sclerosis and all over the world about 2,500,000 sufferers.

The laboratories have the monopoly and they have to sell to Auge, now that the pathology is incorporated in the state as a catastrophic illness. Doses of Interferon, Copaxone or Avonex treatments have an approximate cost of $1,000,000 Chilean pesos a month per person. 3,000 people at $1,000,000 per person = $3,000,000,000 monthly.

Then how much laboratories profit for having us "connected" to these medicines that are only palliative?

We constantly read in newspapers that scientists discover treatments with animals and that they have achieved reverting MS in mice with coffee, or radically improve health of patients with MS using phytotherapy, low fat diets (and I could mention many other treatments), but when these are rejected by medical science, nothing happens and we go back to the same medicine.

What happens with these investigations?

Is there "someone" that silences them?

I am determined to investigate how I can obtain my wellness using alternative media to obtain a better quality of life.

Anything that will make me feel better is welcome. For example, acupuncture, radiostesy, biomagnetism, yoga, reiki, or noesiterapia help us to strengthen physical and spiritually and coexist with our illness.

t This stage and thanks to a visit by my cousin, whom I hadn´t seen in years who made me reconsider a simple question which I hadn´t answered, maybe because I´ve tried to be calm or resigned with the medicine I was subjected.

"What is the composition of myelin? "

Well, from the answer to that question leads to what fats should my body receive in order to help the process of re-myelination.

16. DECIDING TO STOP TAKING MY MEDICINE

On March 27, 2010 I took the decision to suspend my medicine. The pain in my hands, legs and veins was unbearable.

Two or three days later my body started to detoxify and the pain slowly went away. Although I lacked strength and the difficulty of walking remained, it was easier now to do the chores.

Who would have known? And what an irony. The medicine that I went to such pains to get was to blame for my state, for the symptoms had worsened with the medication, or rather I felt worse with it than without it.

G - Water divining (dowsing)

In my yoga classes I began experimenting with dowsing. After my first experience, I felt much better. I had more energy in my legs and I felt different.

Ravi once more was my guide in this new alternative road.

Dowsing (or radiesthésie in French) is a word created in 1920 by the French brothers Bouly. It comes from the Latin word "radius"and the Greek "aistheses "(sensation).

The performer of the Dowsing is the person capable of detecting by means of the pendulum or dowsing wand, the vibrations of stimuli and the radiations issued by things, persons, animals, or lands.

The radiations are issued not only by water and metals, but by any form of life. The dowsing is the study for the investigation of the waves and the vibrations issued by the bodies. The dowsing phenomena have a physical order of explanation: each thing, from inorganic matter to living beings, issue radiations, each with a different wavelength.

The dowser can also detect these wavelengths or natural radiations to find the presence of what he is looking for: ailing of a person, the medicine, therapy or therapeutic support suitable for the cure of the illness and for the holistic cure, water, gold, lost objects, any information on lands.

The Iranian doctor F. Batmanghelidj has performed important studies relating the lack of water in the human body with a list of painful and frequent conditions that overwhelm the individual.

The pathologies of most prevalence for this concept are, among others, the following.

Cerebral sickness (Alzheimer, Parkinson, Multiple Sclerosis...)

Digestive sickness (Gastritis, Heartburn, Constipation...).

Arthritis (Osteoarthritis, Arthritis, Rheumatic Arthritis...)

Lumbago.

Migraine.

Depression, Chronic Fatigue and Stress.

Hypertension

Cholesterol

Overweight

Asthma and Allergies

Diabetes and Dehydration.

The approaches of Dr Batmanghelidj (who I mentioned at the beginning of this book), have raised debate in the scientific and medical world. He pointed out that the prevalence of electromagnetic blockages is accentuated in dehydrated bodies and therefore the intake of at least two litres of water per day is of major importance for good health and wellbeing.

The most ancient traditions of the east had a holistic concept of the human being and considered that illnesses of the body had deeper roots.

Sickness wasn´t for them a lack of energetic harmony in the person. The ancient people seemed to know that all the universe vibrates and is energy.

Each cell and organ of our body vibrates continuously with a pre-determined frequency. When an organ is apparently healthy, its vibratory frequency is in harmony with the rest of the body, but if this frequency is altered the harmony is broken and that is what we call sickness.

H - Healing with the sound of Tibetan bowls and bells

We also know that by this resonance principle, it is possible to modify these altered frequencies through the transmission of other frequencies.

This is what allows sound as a therapeutic process to be

capable of opening the door to physical, emotional, mental and spiritual balance. The sound (frequency) of Tibetan quartz and metallic bowls in harmony with the frequency of the person issued by the bowl can result in both vibrating in the same rhythm.

The quartz bowls induce a frequency of alpha waves that is the same as generated by the brain in the in the meditative and states of profound calm. It has been proved that in these states there is an increased production of T lymphocytes, responsible for the immune system.

My yoga sessions in the company of Tibetan bells began to supply me with additional energy and inner peace, the kind we sometimes need very much.

These sessions reaffirmed my goal of continuing to follow this road and not falling back into the web of conventional treatments.

Months later I heard about a treatment of phytotherapy in Buenos Aires, so I started to investigate again, because I didn´t want another loud mouth filling me with false illusions.

I - Herbal Medicine in Multiple Sclerosis (Phytotherapy)

After studying the topic, I decided to try it. I called Semarmédica in Buenos Aires. The clinic was dedicated to this and I inquired what it is all about. Apparently, it is very interesting - the only problem is that the price is too high.

Well, this doctor has to make a living, I thought.

I asked my friend Bea if she would go with me. I couldn´t travel alone, and she said she would go.

Could I complement this new approach to life that I have proposed using the properties of plants?

Our ancestors used medicinal plants for curing. For many years, plants were the only resource doctors had for healing their patients. They advanced much in their knowledge and they even extracted products from them.

Phytotherapy is the name given to the medicinal use of plants. Many vegetable species used for curing among ancient Egyptians, Greeks, and Romans formed part of the medieval pharmacopeia. Years later they were supplemented with new discoveries from the New World.

At the beginning of this century, the development of chemistry and the discovery of complex processes of organic synthesis started a process on behalf of the pharmaceutical industry of creating new medications. But I still remember what my father used to tell about my grandfather, who was a pharmaceutical chemist. He prepared in his pharmacy the proper medicine for each illness as something unique and personal.

Medicine that is based on medicinal plants has a great advantage compared with chemical concoctions. In plants, active elements are always biologically balanced by the presence of complementary substances that in general don´t accumulate in the system, meaning the unwanted side effects will be limited.

Diseases are the consequence of a large chain of reactions in the human body, due to permanent deteriorating relations with the surrounding microorganisms. It is impossible to defeat sickness if we don´t blend our internal and external factors.

We all participate in one way or another to our state of health or sickness through our beliefs, positive or negative, and our attitude towards life, through the use of therapies we consider adequate for us.

The understanding of this healing process is the first step

towards recuperation.

A malady is not only physical, it is an internal problem inside us. It is not only our physical and mental body, but of our ethereal body (the energies that we have internally).

This combination of body and mind is everything; if it is not working on a healthy path, then our physical part will not improve.

The plants can help us to:

Improve brain circulation.

Reduce depressive symptoms.

Protect eyesight.

Reduce loss of memory.

I can name several plants:

Gingko (Gingko Biloba): Increases blood circulation and is one of the best antioxidants. This has been demonstrated in the treatment of loss of vision, impotency, dizziness, speech problems, lack of memory or concentration.

Passion flower: (Passiflora cacurulea): Effective in the treatment of depressive symptoms and urine incontinence.

Caléndula: (Calendula arvensis): A wonderful wild flower (Calendula officinalis). Effective in loss of muscular mass.

Thyme: (Thymus vulgaris): The same properties as Calendula. Use as thyme oil in compresses, directly on the affected area.

Ginger: (Zingiber officinale): Strong medicine for swelling and is good in the treatment of fatigue. Can be taken as tea or fresh. In Ayurvedic medicine used in India and Chinese medicine it is very important. The Hindu and Chinese cultures used it for millenniums as digestive tea. The Chinese believe it is the yang, or spicy food, which balances the cold food to create harmony. The Greek and Romans also used it for this. It impacted Europe and America as a medicinal herb and became popular as a soft drink (ginger ale, ginger beer and ginger tea) for stomach relief.

Ginger and orange tea with raisins.

Ingredients:

1 orange, 10 raisins, one ginger bulb, honey and water.

Preparation:

Heat 6 cups of water. When it boils add orange in slices with skin, ginger also sliced with skin and raisins. Leave on the side, let stand for 20 minutes, sweeten with honey.

Yogi Tea

This is recommended as a purifier, a toner of the nervous system, liver rebuilder and also for the brain if it has suffered damage by the use of drugs. It helps to balance your system when you feel out of shape. It has been used to prevent colds, sickness of the mucous membrane.

For each cup of tea, add:

300 millilitres of water.

3 cloves

4 Seeds of cardamom

4 grains of black pepper

3 cloves

½ piece of vanilla stick

1 slice of fresh ginger

¼ teaspoon of black tea (optional).

Heat a glass of water, add to previous mixture without letting it boil.

Add half a glass of soy milk for each glass of liquid.

OUR NUTRITION

IS THE FUNDAMENTAL BASE

FOR REGENERATING THE MYELIN

"We are what we eat "

That is why nutrition is so important in the prevention of sickness and if we are already sick, even more so, because we still have time for regenerating our body and produce what we are lacking: Myelin.

According to studies, the countries that consume a greater amount of food rich in saturated fat are the ones that have higher indices of Multiple Sclerosis.

In countries where acid essential fats are consumed in greater quantities, they have smaller numbers of MS patients. This could explain the fact that in the more industrialized countries in the north and centre of Europe and Asia the incidence of this sickness is higher, while in other less industrialized countries it is minor. This would also explain why in Japan, being a more industrialized country, there is a lower occurrence of MS than in Central Europe or the United States due to the great amount of soy or fish in the Japanese diet, food very rich in essential fat acids.

Let´s not be satisfied with conventional medicine. We can try other less aggressive therapies that can be equally or more equally effective.

I am very happy with my yoga routines, Dowsing, Tibetan bowls, all this complemented with an adequate diet and exercise.

I always remember what I should say NO to and to when I should say YES.

NO, to hydrogenated fat found in industrial oils that undergo chemical processes to increase their production and durability at the expense of our health (margarine).

YES, to non-saturated fat, found in Sunflowers (fatty essentials acids) and olive oil (mono-unsaturated) ecological cold pressed.

J - The road to alternative medicine

Yoga is a fundamental part of my existence. The peace and calm that it provides is immense, but even more, it provides the mental clearness in making adequate and assertive decisions.

Thanks to this inner peace I decided to live without chemical medicine, which I had taken during the first sixteen years of my MS.

I could now say NO to the side effects produced by them and which take us nowhere.

I freed myself from the web of the pharmaceutical industry.

It seems that sometimes our vulnerability makes us submit and heed to what the doctors tell us, that the only way is the one full of chemical medicine, but now I am more than sure about this not being the right way.

Sometimes alternative paths can bring more benefit than the traditional medical ways and they help us to get well in another way. As my yoga guide would say, maybe intuition made me look for the road of herbal remedies and natural medicine.

I left for Buenos Aires with Bea, my guardian angel, full of hope for this new therapy they offered.

Doctor Omar Ayrad and his work team helped me to redirect my life and my treatment. They confirmed what I thought about the medication I was submitted to. Not only is it not a cure, but it affects our liver. The cortisone produces a blockage in the production of ACTH of the pituitary glands and the plasmatic Cortizol block the adrenal primary and secondary glands. This appears in the relapses that affect any improvements achieved in my health.

I made important discoveries. Multiple Sclerosis affects both hemispheres of the brain. This creates a lateral curve towards the most affected side, producing pinching of the vertebrae on the nerves. This mostly affects the lumbar and sacral nerves. Of course, I was no exception. A great part of my symptoms was not due to Multiple Sclerosis but to the deviation of my spinal column which was compressing my spinal cord.

The doctor´s herbal treatment consisted of a tea which should be taken in the morning for 6 months. It seems to affect the elimination of the HTLVI, LINPHOTROPI human virus, which apparently is the cause of Multiple Sclerosis. The body auto attacks itself because this virus is located in the myelin. It is defending itself.

This herbal remedy treatment slows down the progress of the sickness and reverses its symptoms, achieving improvement.

I went back to Santiago with six bags of the therapy treatment, concerned about my passing through Chilean customs. it really looked like marihuana in the hands of a Colombian. Fortunately, nothing happened, and Bea and I and the six bags arrived safely home.

I began the treatment for the next six months. Besides

the tea, I also took a miracle "shake" made of cereal, wheat germ, pollen, linseed, sesame seeds, honey and orange juice, and a supplement of vitamins D, B1, B6, B12, Omega 3, coenzyme Q10 and magnesium.

Pollen: This is one of the most complete energizers. The bees extract it from the flowers, make little balls and store them in their combs in small cells specially dedicated for this purpose. This pollen is also fortified with the nectar with which they make honey, which increases its nutrition properties and health benefits. The pollen contains proteins (almost all the essential amino acids), and is a major source of vitamins, minerals and carbohydrates.

Wheat germ: A grain of wheat consists of an external shell, a starchy part and the germ, which is the seed that will grow into the plant. The wheat germ is rich in proteins, vitamins B1, B2, B6, Omega 3, B6 vitamin E and folic acid.

It provides 100% of the magnesium, zinc, copper, molybdenum requirements and an important part of iron and potassium.

Oats: These are one of the cereals most rich in proteins, fat (almost double that of wheat), carbohydrates, vitamin B1 or thiamine (necessary for the proper function of the nervous system). In smaller proportions, oats provide other vitamins from the B group. It contains minerals like phosphorus, potassium, magnesium, calcium and iron.

Sesame: Rich in unsaturated fatty acids, sesame contains 40% linoleic acid or omega 6. The fatty acids - omega 6 especially - play an important part in the balance of the nervous and cardiovascular systems, in the immune defences and also combat the allergic and inflammatory reactions. It's an antioxidant, an excellent source of Vitamin E that helps to prevent the aging of cells and cancer. It is a source of Vitamin B1, involved in the transmission of nervous impulses, and the growth and production of energy.

Remineralizer: This is an excellent source of many minerals and trace elements (iron, calcium, phosphorus, zinc, magnesium, manganese.).

K - The importance of physical exercise

The physical rehabilitation in Multiple Sclerosis is a permanent fight to gain physical condition and fight muscle loss. It is like a relay race where we constantly have to strengthen a different part of our body given that we carry a time bomb inside us.

The important thing is that we keep disciplined and consistent.

It is better to exercise a little, but do it every day, instead of running a marathon in one day. Physical exercise should become a habit. We are the only ones that can do it, nobody else can do it for us. Our rehabilitation is at stake.

It has been demonstrated that a constant physical activity is necessary to avoid complications that can lead to some of the Multiple Sclerosis symptoms and maintain and improve functions that were affected by the illness.

Maybe this is the part that causes most difficulty. It is our neuralgic weak-spot. I know it's not easy to pursue physical exercise when we feel very weak, such as trying to pedal a bicycle. We may finish exhausted, with trembling legs, but we must remember that we need to get strong or else we 'll lose the battle.

When I started exercising again a few months ago, I was too weak to do it, but I knew that it was that, or losing everything. Today, after a few months, I feel stronger. There were days when I had to lie down after I had been on the bike for a few minutes. There is a saying that being constant gets you what you couldn´t get easily and for that I thank my yoga teacher and Sergio for encouraging me to be consistent in my physical efforts.

Every person with MS, no matter how severe their disability, should exercise regularly. The lack of exercise can be the cause of serious health consequences. Exercise not only provides a sensation of well-being - it is also important in the prevention of future problems.

Exercises can be divided in five categories:

- **To acquire flexibility** - This implies the stretching of muscles and tendons with the mobility of the joints. These activities prevent the reduction of mobility, stiffness, weakness and spasticity.

- **To fortify** - Increase your muscle strength. These can be fortified with the use of an elastic band, lifting weights, even pushing against a wall.

- **Gaining resistance** - Increasing resistance will reduce the risk of heart problems, regulate cholesterol levels and maintaining the right weight. Walk, swim, ride a static bike, are some of the physical activities that increase resistance.

- **Balance and Coordination** - Helps the quality and assurance of our movements. Rhythmic exercise of the hands and feet with certain specific activities, preferably supervised, can improve balance and coordination.

- **Relaxation** - Reduces physical and mental tension. A program of structured relaxation can relieve fatigue after exercising sessions. It can also help in getting through a day full of tension.

17. OUR TRAVELING COMPANIONS

In this stage of this book I want to reflect on those people who are with us day by day in our struggle (husbands, wives, partners, parents, sons, relations, friends) that are near us when we get sick and helpless. They form a fundamental part of our recovery.

Their lives have also changed significantly, having to assume different tasks they didn´t have to do before.

Sometimes when a person has a physical impairment they tend to think that it limits their own abilities and thoughts. Sometimes the one suffering the illness feels left aside, thinking that their opinions are permanently on vacation and that they are unwittingly excluded, often in critical decisions that have to be taken.

The work of taking care of a patient with a degenerative illness can be difficult, because as time passes, the patient stops doing things they did before without even noticing.

With degenerative illness, little by little the acts such as dressing, walking, bathing may become progressively limited. This can create an unintended dependency on the person who is near to us.

We can make life difficult for them as the home environment becomes more complicated. We must understand that we, the patients, have to notice when our carers are stressed or in a bad humour.

And in turn, our carer should understand how important it is to keep on pushing the patient, for this can give the patient a sense of their own value.

I understand that in the long run some illnesses can also affect the mental faculties of a person, but I am sure that if the relation of the patient with those who surround them is close, this process will be delayed and probably won´t reach this regrettable state.

That´s why I can offer some advice that may help you:

- Control your temper.

- Create tasks for both parties

- Avoid saying: I can´t or you can´t. If possible, rather say: I will try.

- Consider the other person and think "if I were you, what would I do".

- Take time to think before you talk, in case you say something you might regret later. Words don't come back after you have said them.

- In a healthy and busy mind, there is no room for blame recriminations.

18. CONLCUSIONS

When I began writing this book, I didn´t imagine that the answer I was looking for was within myself. I looked for the changes I needed to make and the reasons for making them so I could pursue them in order to reach my successful healing.

I can´t deny that what I have learned in these eighteen years is marvellous. I have discovered very interesting things, but especially in these last two years when I finally did find what every patient looks for: their definite healing and inner peace.

Important topics like stress, good nutrition or rather the appropriate nutrition according to our needs, the advantages of water and its healing properties, the power of good music, of good company, importance of daily exercise, banishing things that don´t agree with me, the advantages of a good relaxation technique like yoga, building my energy levels, the curing and healing properties of food and plants... I could go on and on mentioning many more.

But for this healing process to happen there must be a radical change inside us.

Our attitude towards life and our illness - we must accept our condition and be positive that we will accomplish this and win the healing battle.

We can use the wonderful energy of our body and it can make us heal. The miracle happens within us. I am convinced that when people heal, they have been through those stages that make their total healing possible. That is why we sometimes hear of people who attend a healing mass and come out cured. It's simply that their mind is so powerful that they believe they can be cured and in a positive way they achieve this.

As for myself, I feel different. After being a total invalid, depending on a wheelchair, without being able to dress myself alone, I began to believe in myself. Miracles happen, **we** make them possible. I still get around with two crutches and when I go to a mall I use a wheelchair. But now I don´t care, I know that God stowed this ordeal upon me, but I´m sure he wouldn´t have put a heavier burden on my shoulders if I couldn´t carry it. I accepted my illness, I enjoy every day and I think I am fortunate in being able to do this and be with my loved ones.

I don´t know if I will ever walk again, but I know that my mind now can see things under a different perspective, that of a person who is more calm, serene, that thinks positively. The rest is in God´s hands and the universe.

"When you want something, all the universe conspires for your wish to come through." Paulo Cohelho.

The real healing starts by giving us the tools and through our consciousness we heal, not only through our rational consciousness, but through our own feelings and affection.

Bruce Lipton, speaking of the power of our mind, says that you can change the chemistry of the mind, the epigenetic control (above that of the genes) and achieve a change that can heal a sickness. The genes, as he says, are controlled by the subconscious, which is a machine that reprograms itself with all the experiences one has had. It is here where daily reality enters. He also believes that the mind of the patient is two-thirds of the control of the healing process.

We have to make decisions. The function of the mind is to create coherence between what we really believe and our reality.

The less we know about the bad part of what ails us, the better we trust what we can achieve. He refers to a phrase from Albert Einstein: *"The most important decision we can make in our lives is to decide once and for all if we live in a hostile and negative universe or in one that is friendly and supportive."*

We have been made to believe that we can´t cure ourselves and that it is the doctors who have the healing power.

Let´s remember Deepak Chopra who talks about the power of the intention or strength that allows if we want to heal. First, we need clarity and we must feel it in our consciousness. The healing force is in ourselves; all we need is to guide our imagination to reach it. We are connected with everything that happens in the universe.

The universe will conspire again and again until it enables you to fulfil the purpose of your change of life. We must be attentive to all its manifestations, even the smallest ones because from each one we will get something positive so we can advance to conquer the problem. Whatever doesn´t help us - the negatives (work, people, attitudes) we should cast aside so they can´t either affect or harm us. These negatives might make us believe that we won´t be capable of conquering our goal.

"When you lose contact with your inner peace, you lose contact with yourself, you get lost in the world. Your most inner feeling of yourself, the sense of who you are is inseparable from peace. That is the I am, which is deeper than names and forms. Inner peace is your essential nature." (Eckhart Tolle).

AKNOWLEDGEMENTS

To Sergio, Laura, Juan Pablo and Daniel for supporting me every day, for being my legs when I didn´t have them, for helping me with the daily chores when I couldn´t, for making me laugh when I was sad and depressed, for boosting me to continue my battle and return to the path, in short, for being the light in my life and the reason of my existence.

To my friend, Beatriz Podestá, for giving me back my self-esteem and the eagerness to continue fighting, for sharing her twinkling and positive spirit with me in the most difficult moments of my life, for being the sister I never had and the accomplice in all my adventures, for inviting me to share with her a bit of her daily life.

To all my friends, for encouraging in me the desire to struggle, recover happiness, and the thought that IT IS POSSIBLE TO DEFEAT AN IMPOSSIBLE.

To Ravi Kaur Khalsa for giving me strength and inner peace through yoga, necessary for healing, for her weekly dedication with me in a disinterested way. For teaching me that I could be my own healer, simply with a positive attitude toward life and my own illness, by listening to my inner silence and the messages that my own body was giving me.

To all those who helped me in different ways to withdraw my economic stress, which would never let my body heal. Especially Tomás Cox and Patricia Ready, for their constant concern towards me, my family and their help.

To my parents for giving me life, for teaching me all they could and gauging what was right for me. For having fought tirelessly in giving me the best of childhoods.

APPENDIX I - MULTIPLE SCLEROSIS DIET

I have summarized the diet I have been on for 18 years, which I have improved and I can say now that thanks to it I have kept my sclerosis more or less stable all these years.

I hope my experience can help others.

Originally, I started with Doctor Ray Lavender Swank´s and Barbara Brewer Dugan´s diet, but in the long run I noticed that it was too easy in some aspects and on the other hand after much self-experimentation I discovered food that was very important for the stability of my system. I wound up relying on what we could call vegetarian but with a high content of fish: mackerel, tuna, bonito, salmon, tooth fish, anchovies, shrimp and egg whites.

Exclude from the diet: milk and any of its processed derivatives, sausages, octopus, squid, fried food, mayonnaise, beef, pork, saturated fat, egg yolks, cookies, packaged potato chips, chocolate, soft drinks, coconut, palm oil, coconut oil.

Use olive oil always, which should be kept in the refrigerator as heat destroys vitamin E which is an antioxidant and which protects olive oil from becoming musty (changes in odour and flavour).

Remove from the diet prepared products like crackers, biscuits, fried potatoes, doughnuts, garbage food, packaged soup, because they all contain hydrogenated oils, generally palm and coconut oil.

Eliminate red meat, pork, sausages, hams, foie gras.

The use of sugar is not restricted but it is better to use brown sugar. My experience is that honey is much better for the healing properties it has.

In case we need chocolate for brownies or a cake it would be better to use chocolate syrup or cocoa as they don´t contain fat.

Beverages: No alcohol. (In special occasions a glass of red wine is all right).

Limit the use of sodas and energizers.

Moderate use of: Tea and coffee (2 or 3 cups a day).

Advisable foods:

Fresh fruit juice, green tea, ginger tea and cinnamon, yogic tea, tisanes.

Soy in all its forms: Beans, mashed, steak, milk, juice, tofu.

Nuts and dried fruit, walnuts, almonds, sesame seed, linseed, raisins, peaches, pineapple, dehydrated apple, ginger, cinnamon.

Salmon, mackerel, anchovies, tuna, trout, whitefish, tooth fish, conger eel, and in general any other salt water fish and white meat.

Shell fish, crab, prawn, shrimp, lobster, mussels, clams.

Sometimes octopus and squid are excluded from the diet and that people with high levels of cholesterol must be careful with shell fish.

Vegetables

Especially the greens, broccoli, cauliflower, asparagus, spinach, lettuce, cabbage, celery, Italian pumpkin, avocado, Brussel sprouts, cucumber, pimento, carrots, onion.

In all the diets, especially in Doctor Swank's, it is recommended that you not over-indulge in fruit and vegetables with a high percentage of unsaturated fat like avocado and olives.

Fruit

They are all good for your health, but I would say that there is a vital one. BANANA. Eating one or two bananas a day can regulate our mood and provide necessary energy. Melon, strawberries, cranberries, apples, pears, bananas, oranges, lemons, tangerines, peaches, grapes, plums.

Eggs

Egg whites can be included without any restriction. The white of an egg contains three grams of protein and no fat.

Grains

Wheat, soy, rice, cereal and whole wheat cereals, lentils, pasta, beans, chick beans, peas (and potatoes) can be eaten with no restriction (remember, that grains have to be soaked in water from one day to another, as the protein, which is hard, will soften when cooking). Brewers' yeast, wheat germ, or soy lecithin are excellent alternatives.

Choose black bread, water biscuits or rice, whole wheat bread over white bread.

APPENDIX II - VITAMINS AND SUPPLEMENTS

In an article published in the American Medical Association Journal, December 20, 2006, members of the Public Health School of Harvard University and the Department of Molecular Biology, University of South Carolina, intend to study if levels of the 25-hydrovitamin D are associated with the risk of developing Multiple Sclerosis.

Vitamin D is a strong modulator of the immune response. Multiple Sclerosis is an auto immune sickness, in which unknown agents start up an inflammatory response, through T lymphocytes, which causes the loss of myelin (demyelization) in the central nervous system.

High levels of vitamin D circulating in the blood are associated with a minor risk of Multiple Sclerosis.

Vitamins of the B group.

The vitamins of the B group have great influence on the performance of the brain and the nervous system.

B1 or thiamine.

Thiamine plays a fundamental part in the metabolism of

carbon hydrates. Its lack affects the tissues that depend most on this energetic supplement, like the brain. The lack of this vitamin produces loss of concentration and memory and can be the cause of depression. We find it in fresh soy, wheat germ, fish, dry fruit (Brazil nuts), vegetables or integral cereals, especially oats.

B6 or pyridoxine.

This is involved in several aspects of metabolism and the biosynthesis of several neurotransmitters, including the serotonin coming from tryptophan and the formation of the myelin sheath of the neurons - isolation needed for the correct transmission of signals via the nerve fibres. This is how the brain sends instructions to the muscles of our body. Its deficient input can be the cause of irritability, nervousness, fatigue, and depression. We find this vitamin in wheat germ, blue fish, dried fruit, integral oats, vegetables and brewer yeast.

Vitamin B 12

Involved in the proper performance of the nervous system, its deficiency causes neurologic alterations, such as sensitive neuropathy, resulting in irritability and depression. Foods of animal origin is the dietetic source of this vitamin, such as blue fish (sardines) and eggs.

Vitamin E.

I found a very simple medicine to obtain vitamin E: Avocado. It is adequate for stress conditions and low defences. Recent investigations carried out by UCLA show that avocado has more vitamin E than any other fruit. From a nutritional point of view, it contains many vitamins and photo chemical substances, which help protect the body from sickness.

Linseed

Only in linseed do we find essential acids perfectly balanced. Reports published by the Karolinske Institute in Switzerland show that linseed contains 800mg/kg of essential acids.

The lignin in linseed (anti-cancer agents) contain 100 times more properties than the best integral grains. They help in preventing breast and colon cancer. Simply add a teaspoon of ground linseed to your diet.

A spoonful of linseed also contains more than 800 mg of ALNA, the primary acid fat Omega 3. Linseed his is 10 times more ALNA than the majority of fish oils. without the consequences such as fish flavour, the level of cholesterol and the high levels of saturated fats in fish oils.

All the fatty essential acids are necessary for human health. These acids can´t be manufactured in the body and should be included in our daily diet.

In addition, linseed fibre is known for its capability to 'smooth' the large intestine, preventing constipation. Mucilage (soluble fibre) is a mucous substance that is found under the skin of the seed and has the property of blocking the excess of acid. It acts like a natural laxative, protecting the delicate bowel without side effects. The soluble fibre of linseed prevents the absorption of cholesterol in food, and increases the amount that is excreted by the system. The mucilage of the lint helps the stabilizing and modulating of blood glucose.

Its oils are high quality, but when they are ground and turned into flour, these oils decompose very rapidly.

In the context of feeding the world, linseed should be an important element for greater mental and physical development.

Omega 3

The body needs the acid fat omega 3 (linoleic acid) to function correctly. Among the main functions of linoleic acid, the following can be found.

The formation of hormones.

The correct function of the immunological system.

The correct formation of the retina.

The correct function of neurons and chemical transmissions.

Magnesium

Magnesium is almost a miraculous mineral for its healing effect on a great variety of sicknesses as well as its capacity in rejuvenating the ageing body. It is well known that it is essential for many enzyme reactions, especially in those related to the production of cellular energy, for brain health, the nervous system and also for teeth and bone health.

Q10 coenzyme

The coenzymes are essential molecules that make it possible for our body to work in a more efficient way.

Coenzyme Q10 helps the generation of energy. Even if the body can get all the raw materials needed for obtaining the mentioned energy, it is not enough if the transforming mechanism doesn´t work correctly. It needs a "spark" that starts the process of converting food into energy. Without the Q10 coenzyme, the spark can´t be produced, nor the energy.

Q10 is necessary for the transformation and contribution of energy to living cells.

In allergic processes, sometimes the Q10 coenzyme helps as a natural antihistamine.

Coenzyme Q10 strengthens the immune system. It increases the physiological capacity of the use of oxygen, particularly in stress situations and supports the function of the immunological system.

Coenzyme Q10 increases longevity by delaying aging. This is due to its antioxidant power, neutralizing free radicals. Its antioxidant action is similar to that of vitamins E and K – it inhibits the cellular destruction induced by free radicals by neutralizing them through oxygenating reactions.

Patients with muscular dystrophy seem to possess reduced levels of coenzyme Q10. Supplementation with coenzyme Q10 can improve their quality of life.

A dosage of 1 milligram is recommended for each pound of an individual's weight.

Relaxants

For combating excess nervousness, make sure that the nervous system is well nourished including food mentioned earlier (carbon hydrates, tryptophan, vitamins of group B, iron and phospholipids). It is advisable to include integral foods, cereals like oats, dry fruit, vegetables, seed oil, and diet complements such as brewer's yeast, wheat grain, soy lecithin, wheat, orange blossom, espino albar, melissa, passion flower, valerian, tila.

Dangerous food:

Aspartame (Nutra Sweet)

The intake of aspartame has been indicated as a possible cause of Multiple Sclerosis, although critics argue that they do not support this position and that the product has no relation with any illness. Just in case I banished aspartame, replacing it with other sweeteners like honey and brown sugar.

Appendix III - TWO POSSIBLE ALTERNATIVE THERAPIES DIFFERENT FROM THOSE I USED.

L - Bio-magnetism

This consists of the recognition of altered energy spots in our system that together are giving cause to an acute or chronic illness. This process is carried out using passive magnets (not electrified nor connected to electronic machines). The magnets are applied to various zones of the body, like a bio-magnetic scanner. Once the altered zones are recognized and confirmed in their energetic potential (and correspond with organs and tissues that are distorted), the therapist applies various magnets in those spots for times that vary between 10 and 15 minutes for each. In general, they are applied simultaneously.

We should remember that all beings are kept healthy when there is an energetic balance in our systems, organs and tissues. This balance is made by a delicate and complex structure of cells that are constantly exchanging information between themselves. In turn, the cells require the right environment to keep functioning correctly. This is of vital importance for the ionic balance in them and their environment. There are positive and negative charges, giving a balance between acid and basic charges. or balance of pH. The human body keeps in good health if its pH or internal acidity is maintained at a neutral zone close to pH 7.

When something is altered, whether by virus, bacteria, toxicity or fungus, an alteration in its acidity or pH is produced and the cells involved are altered in their performance. This damages their proper function, and at the same time promotes the feeding of the problem (the bacteria, virus, fungus, parasite etc.). The illness or alteration of a part of the body needs the distortion or lack of balance between positive and negative charges to remain so it can continue as a problem. If the ionic alteration is fixed and balanced, the problem disappears.

The bio-magnetism takes care of this. Thanks to the magnet's strength it is capable of impacting a similar pathologic polarity and makes it balance with its similar opposite polarity, thus neutralising them, making their value zero.

Several sessions are needed for correcting the changes that cause illnesses like HIV, Multiple Sclerosis, Cirrhosis, Fibromyalgia, Diabetes, Syphilis, TBC, Coronary, Nephritis, Hepatitis, Cancer, Asthmatic processes.

Dr Madeleine F. Barnothi, physics professor at the University of Illinois, defines Bio-magnetism as the science of the processes and induced functions through a magnetic static field in live organs.

Dr Howard D. Strangle of New York considers that magnetism is a real science and states that it is a topic that should awaken world interest.

Dr Samuel Hahnemann (1755-1843), founder and teacher of Homeopathy, in his Medical Homeopathic Organon, asserts that a magnetized bar can cure fast and permanently the most severe of the diseases for which it is the appropriate medicine.

M - Acupuncture

I have heard from colleagues that acupuncture is a valid tool in recovery.

MS is characterized by an important energetic deficiency. The function of the acupuncture therapist is to maintain an energetic tone in the patient, both nutritive and emotional.

The wear on the body of MS requires a permanent enrichment of the patient in dietetic level, supplements, acupuncture and healthy life habits.

Among the symptoms there could be muscular atrophy, optic nerve atrophy, paralysis, dizziness, aphasia, loss of vision, depression, anxiety, allergies, etc.

The loss of the immunological system must be avoided, to prevent organic and mental damage.

The brain and the medulla need nutrients for maintaining the level of energy and blood in an optimum state.

The factors of humidity-heat is harmful for an MS sufferer, as it breaches the cerebral and medullar functions

Intense heat damages the mobilization functions and transformation of liquids and nutrients, blocking the blood flow and energy.

When the body suffers damage at an organic level, the first organ affected is the kidney. This organ exhausts the body's essential energy. The deficiency of the Yin exhausts the basal Jing, by not allowing the nutrition in bones, medulla, tendons and muscles. In turn, this can generate stiffness and painful paralysis.

The wind ascends to cephalic level causing an elevation of the Yang because of the deficiency of the Yin and as it bothers the cephalic level, causing dizziness.

The illness in its evolution extends its symptoms, like the deficiency of the kidney's Yang, revealing itself through hypothermia, urinary frequency and incontinence.

The loss of Qi produces exhaustion in the spleen and pancreas, limiting the amount and quality in the blood and so limiting the tendon-muscular nutrition.

The liver, feeling attacked by the insufficiency of the

Yin, causes anxiety, irritability and blockage of energy. As the liver can´t nurture the brain, it causes blood stasis blockage of the Qi and damages the cardiac functions. The patient loses quality of life in their personal and social relations, suffering a decrease in libido, crying and depression.

The optical treatment of MTC should be done at the beginning of the medical history of the patient. Treatment for the heat symptoms, humidity, wind, deficiency of Qi, Yin and Yang, also tone the Jing and the Qi.

Acupuncture will decrease the medication until it disappears if it is accompanied by diet and orthomol supplements, eliminating the corticosteroids. Massages are advisable and also a quiet and pleasant experience and daily exercise. Analytical monitoring and diet are most important for controlling the blood nutrients.

The diet, in the process the individual is going through, must be adapted to the predominance of the symptoms. If these are of humidity in the diet, the humid elements should be abolished. If the symptom is heat you have to cool the Xue; if there is insufficient Yang, provide more Yin.

The supplements must be personalized according to the illness. If there is pain it will be better to be on an antalgic diet with supplemental oligoelements and antioxidants, anti-flammatories and regenerators of the nervous sheath.

REFERENCES

- Almudena Reguero. Periodista especializada en salud y terapias naturales. http://www.alimentacion-sana.com

- Concha Martínez. Homeopatía según diferenciación de síndromes.

- Cousins, Norman. Anatomía de una enfermedad o la voluntad de vivir. KAIROS 1982.

- Dr Samuel Hahnemann (1755-1843). Organón Médico Homeopático

- Dr. Ángel Escudero. Curación por el pensamiento (Noesiterapia). http://dr.escudero.com/libro.html

- Eckhart Tolle. Quietud interior

- Erasmus V. Falts and Olis, Vancouver. La Linaza.; Alive Books, 1986.

- F. Batmanghelidj, M.D. Your Body's Many Cries for Water.

- Federación Española para la lucha contra la Esclerosis Múltiple. Ejercicios de fisioterapia.

- George Bernard Shaw

- Ginger (UCLA). Medical plants, herbs

- http://personal.redestb.es/martin/PFITO.HTM

- http://www.universoyoga.com

- Joan Borysenko MD. Tu Mente Puede Curarte.

- Jorge Correale, jefe de neuro-inmunología de Fleni, revista Brain "la deficiencia de vitamina D se asocia con un mayor riesgo de esclerosis múltiple".

- José N. Dekovic Torres

- Luz Adriana Neira - María Ninelly Neira. Terapia de la risa para nuestros niños hospitalizados. Fundación Doctora Clown.1999. Colombia

- Mario Benedetti. Poema No te rindas.

- Masaru Emoto. Mensajes del agua.

- Pablo Coelho. El Alquimista.

- Revista, consumer.es/web/es/20051001/alimentación/

- Rhonda Byrne. El Secreto.

- Sanación Cuántica del Hospital Haldein

- Santiago Rojas Posada. La estrategia del Ave Fénix. Editorial Norma.

- Sebastián A. Ríos. LA NACION. Vitamina D

- Semarmedica. Pack de información entregado al enfermo con esclerosis múltiple.

- TANTRA. La sexualidad sagrada. http://tantra.fiestras.com

www.ingramcontent.com/pod-product-compliance
Lightning Source LLC
Chambersburg PA
CBHW020325290526
45785CB00007B/2926